5 Ingredients Pressure Cooker Cookbook

Quick and Easy Recipes for Fast and Healthy Meals

W0006215

Maria Marshal

Table Of Contents

BREAKFAST
RECIPES
Vegan Cranberry Oatmeal
(Ready in about 15 minutes | Servings 2)

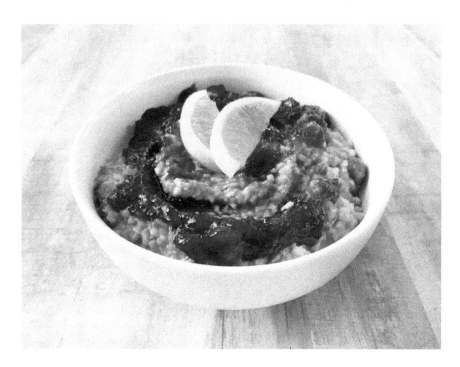

Ingredients

1. 3 cups water

1. 1 cup steel-cut oats

1. 2 teaspoons vegan margarine

1. 1 cup apple juice

1. 4 tablespoons dried cranberries

1. 1-2 tablespoons brown sugar

1. 1/4 teaspoon cardamom

1. 1/4 teaspoon ground cinnamon

Directions

1. Place a metal rack in the pressure cooker; pour in 1/2 cup of water.

2. Add all the above ingredients to a metal bowl that fits inside the pressure cooker. Stir to combine.

3. Cover and bring to LOW pressure. Then, maintain pressure for 8 minutes.

4. Next, allow pressure to release naturally. Serve right away!

Maple Apple Oatmeal

(Ready in about 15 minutes | Servings 2)

Ingredients

1. 3⁄4 cup water

1. 1 cup milk

1. 2 tablespoons dried apricots

1. 1 apple, cored and diced

1. 1 cup toasted quick-cooking oats

1. 2 tablespoons maple syrup

1. 2 tablespoons walnuts, chopped

Directions

1. Simply throw all the above ingredients into your pressure cooker.

2. Now lock the lid into place. Then, maintain HIGH pressure for 5 minutes.

3. Next, remove the cooker from the heat; allow pressure to release. Serve right now and enjoy!

Sausage Breakfast Casserole

(Ready in about 15 minutes | Servings 4)

Ingredients

1. 2 tablespoons canola oil

1. 1 yellow onion, diced

1. 1 small-sized red bell pepper, seeded and chopped

1. 1/2 pound sausage

1. 3 cups potatoes, shredded

1. 6 eggs, beaten

1. 1 cup Ricotta cheese

1. 2 cups Cheddar cheese

1. 3/4 teaspoon salt

1. 1/4 teaspoon ground black pepper

Directions

1. Warm canola oil in the pressure cooker; now sauté the onion and bell pepper until they are tender. Add the sausage and cook for about 3 moreminutes.

2. Add the remaining ingredients to the pressure cooker. Lock the lid intoplace; then, maintain HIGH pressure for about 5 minutes.

3. Remove from the heat. Serve warm and enjoy!

Mom's Berry Jam

(Ready in about 1 hour 20 minutes |
Servings 16)

Ingredients

1. 1 pound raspberries

1. 1 pound blackberries

1. 1 vanilla bean, halved lengthwise

1. 1 ½ pounds honey

Directions

1. Throw all the above ingredients into your pressure cooker. Now place thecooker over medium-high heat, bring it to a boil; stir often.

2. Cover and bring it to pressure. Next, lower the heat to medium-low for 10minutes. Allow pressure to release naturally.

3. Uncover the pressure cooker and place it back on medium-high heat; bringto a boil for 4 to 5 minutes, stirring frequently.

4. Lastly, ladle your jam into hot sterilized jars. Seal the jars. Serve withEnglish muffins if desired. Enjoy!

Old-Fashioned Grits

(Ready in about 15 minutes | Servings 4)

Ingredients

1. 4 cups water

1. A pinch of salt

1. 1/4 teaspoon grated nutmeg

1. 1 cup stone-ground grits

1. 1 tablespoon ghee

Directions

1. Bring the water, salt, and nutmeg to a boil in your pressure cooker overHIGH heat.

2. Gradually stir in the grits and lock the lid into place. Bring to high pressureover high heat; maintain pressure for 10 minutes.

3. Allow steam to release naturally. Lastly, stir in ghee just before serving.Serve and enjoy!

FAST SNACKS RECIPES
Jalapeño and Cheese Dip
(Ready in about 10 minutes | Servings 12)

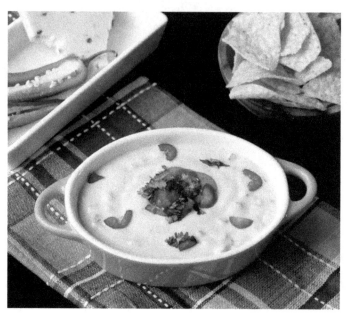

Ingredients

1. 2 tablespoons butter

1. 2 tablespoons all-purpose flour

1. 1 cup milk

1. 16 ounces Monterey Jack cheese, shredded

1. 2 pickled jalapeños, minced

1. 1/2 cup tomatoes, canned

1. 1/4 teaspoon black pepper

1. 1/4 teaspoon cayenne pepper

1. 1 teaspoon basil

1. Sea salt, to taste

Directions

1. In your cooker, warm the butter over medium flame; slowly stir in the flourand stir until you have a paste. Pour in the milk and stir until the mixture has thickened. Bring it to a boil.

2. Add the cheese; vigorously stir until it is smooth. Add the rest of your ingredients; secure the lid on your cooker. Cook on medium; lower heat andcook for about 3 minutes.

3. Afterwards, remove the lid and serve right away.

BBQ Chicken Wings
(Ready in about 25 minutes | Servings 6)

Ingredients

1. 12-15 chicken wings (about 2 pounds)

1. 1/2 teaspoon ground black pepper

1. 1 teaspoon cayenne pepper

1. 1 ¼ teaspoons salt

1. 2 tablespoons olive oil

1. 3 cloves garlic, minced

1. 1 yellow onion, chopped

1. 1/4 cup flour

1. 1/2 cup BBQ Sauce

Directions

1. Season chicken wings with black pepper, cayenne pepper, and salt.

2. Warm olive oil and sauté the garlic and yellow onion. Stir in seasonedchicken wings and cook until they are browned.

3. Then, dust the chicken wings with flour. Pour in the BBQ sauce. Place the lid on your cooker and lock the lid. Press the "Soup/Stew", and cook for 15minutes. Release the pressure value to open.

4. Lastly, test the chicken wings for the doneness. Taste and adjust the seasonings. Serve warm.

Hot Party Wings

(Ready in about 20 minutes | Servings 6)

Ingredients

1. 1 cup water

1. 2 pounds chicken wings

1. 4 tablespoons hot sauce

1. 1/4 cup honey

1. 1/4 cup tomato paste

1. 1 teaspoon ground black pepper

1. 1 teaspoon dried basil

1. 2 teaspoons sea salt

Directions

1. Pour the water into your pressure cooker; place a steamer basket in thecooker.

2. Place the wings in the steamer basket. Close and lock the cooker's lid.Cook for 10 minutes at HIGH pressure.

3. While the chicken wings are cooking, prepare the dipping sauce by mixingthe hot sauce, honey, tomato paste, black pepper, basil, and salt.

4. Then, open the cooker by releasing the pressure. Transfer the prepared wings to the bowl with sauce and coat them evenly. Cook under the broilerfor about 5 minutes, until they become crisp. Enjoy!

Beets with Walnuts

(Ready in about 15 minutes | Servings 6)

Ingredients

1. 6 medium-sized beets

1. 2 ½ cups water

1. 1 tablespoon apple cider vinegar

1. 1 tablespoon honey

1. 1/2 teaspoon paprika

1. 1 teaspoon dried basil

1. 1/2 teaspoon freshly ground black pepper

1. 3/4 teaspoon salt

1. 3 tablespoons extra-virgin olive oil

1. 2 tablespoons walnuts, finely chopped

Directions

1. Scrub your beets. Transfer them to a pressure cooker; pour in the water. Close the cooker's lid and bring to HIGH pressure. Reduce heat to medium;cook for 10 minutes.

2. Remove from heat and release pressure through the steam vent. Remove thelid. Drain the beets and let them cool. Then, rub off skins and cut into wedges. Transfer them to a serving bowl.

3. Whisk the vinegar, honey, paprika, basil, black pepper, salt, and olive oil ina small-sized bowl. Drizzle the vinaigrette over the beets in the serving bowl. Scatter chopped walnuts over the top and serve.

Beets and Carrots with Pecans

(Ready in about 15 minutes | Servings 6)

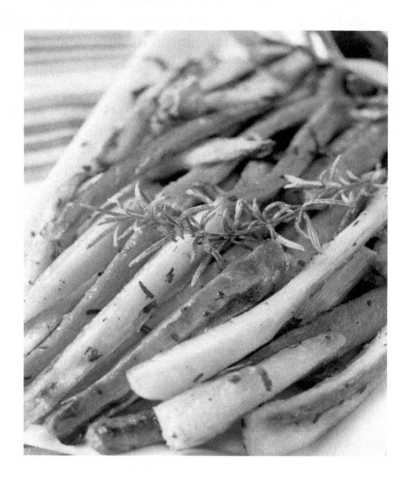

Ingredients

1. 2 ½ cups water

1. 4 medium-sized beets, peeled

1. 4 carrots, trimmed

1. 1 tablespoon fresh lemon juice

1. 1 tablespoon maple syrup
1. 1 teaspoon cumin

1. 1 teaspoon dried dill weed

1. 1 teaspoon salt

1. 1/2 teaspoon freshly ground black pepper

1. 3 tablespoons extra-virgin olive oil

1. 2 tablespoons pecans, finely chopped

1. 2 tablespoons golden raisins

Directions

1. Place water, beets, and carrots in your pressure cooker. Close the lid andbring to HIGH pressure. Now cook for 10 minutes.

2. Turn off the heat and release pressure through steam vent. Drain and rinsebeets and carrots. Cut them into wedges and replace to a bowl in order to cool completely.

3. In a mixing bowl or a measuring cup, whisk the lemon juice, maple syrup,cumin, dill, salt, black pepper, and olive oil.

4. Drizzle the dressing over the vegetables. Scatter pecans and raisins over thetop and serve.

LUNCH RECIPES
Delicious Pea and Ham Soup
(Ready in about 30 minutes | Servings 8)

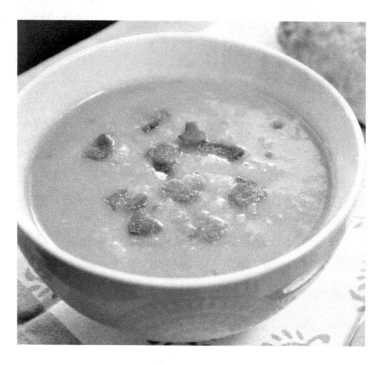

Ingredients

1. 1 pound dried split peas

1. 8 cups water

1. 1 ham bone

1. 1 cup scallions, chopped

1. 2 carrots, diced

1. 2 parsnips, diced

1. 1 teaspoon mustard seed

1. 1 teaspoon dried basil

1. 2 tablespoons sherry wine

Directions

1. Fill the pressure cooker with all the above ingredients, except for sherry wine.

2. Put the lid on your pressure cooker, and bring to HIGH pressure. Cook for20 minutes.

3. Add sherry and stir to combine. Serve and enjoy!

Easiest Adzuki Beans Ever

(Ready in about 10 minutes | Servings 4)

Ingredients

1. 4 cups water

1. 1 cup adzuki beans

1. 2 tablespoons canola oil

1. 1/2 teaspoon black pepper, ground

1. 1 teaspoon salt

1. 1 bay leaf

Directions

1. Fill the pressure cooker with all the above ingredients.

2. Seal the lid; bring to HIGH pressure and maintain for 8 minutes.

3. Then, allow pressure to release naturally. Ladle into soup bowls and servehot.

Black Bean Salad

(Ready in about 10 minutes + chilling time | Servings 6)

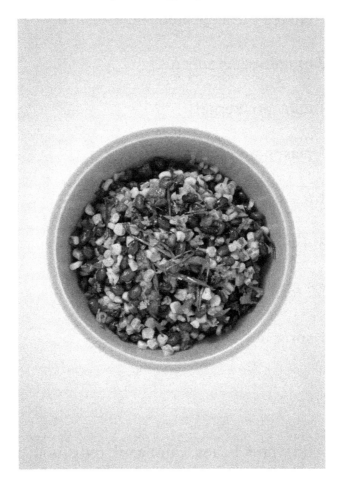

Ingredients

1. 4 cups water

1. 2 cups black beans, soaked overnight

1. 1 tablespoon canola oil

1. 1 red onion, chopped

1. 2 cloves garlic, peeled and smashed

1. 2 tomatoes, chopped

1. 1 cup corn kernels

1. 3 teaspoons olive oil

1. 1 teaspoon apple cider vinegar

1. 3/4 teaspoon salt

1. 1/2 teaspoon white pepper

1. 1 sprig fresh thyme

Directions

1. Add water, beans, canola oil, red onion, and garlic to the pressure cooker.Now lock the lid.

2. Turn the heat to HIGH; cook approximately 8 minutes.

3. Next, wait for the pressure to come down.

4. Strain the beans and transfer them to a refrigerator in order to cool completely. Transfer to a serving bowl and add the rest of the ingredients.Enjoy!

Easiest Pinto Beans Ever

(Ready in about 1 hour 15 minutes |
Servings 6)

Ingredients

1. 8 cups water

1. 1 cup dried pinto beans

1. 2 tablespoons canola oil

1. 2 bay leaves

1. 1 teaspoon salt

1. 3/4 teaspoon ground black pepper

Directions

1. Add 4 cups of water and pinto beans to your pressure cooker. Cover withthe lid and bring to HIGH pressure for 1 minute. Then, quick-release the pressure.

2. Drain and rinse the beans; add the beans back to the pressure cooker. Letthem soak for about 1 hour.

3. Add the rest of the ingredients; bring to HIGH pressure and maintain for about 11 minutes. Serve warm and enjoy!

Yellow Lentil with Kale

(Ready in about 25 minutes | Servings 4)

Ingredients

1. 1 tablespoon canola oil

1. 1 medium-sized leek, diced

1. 1/4 teaspoon coriander

1. 1/2 teaspoon thyme

1. 1/4 teaspoon cumin

1. 1 cup yellow dried lentils

1. 2 tomatoes, chopped

1. 1/2 cup water

1. 2 cups kale, torn into small pieces

Directions

1. Heat canola oil in your pressure cooker over medium heat. Sauté the leeks together with coriander, thyme, and cumin for about 5 minutes. Then, addlentils, tomatoes, and water; stir well to combine. Close and lock the pressure cooker's lid.

2. Cook for about 12 minutes at HIGH pressure.

3. Afterwards, release the pressure according to manufacturer's instructions.Mix in the kale; stir until it is wilted; serve.

DINNER RECIPES
Tomato and Eggplant Salad
(Ready in about 15 minutes | Servings 6)

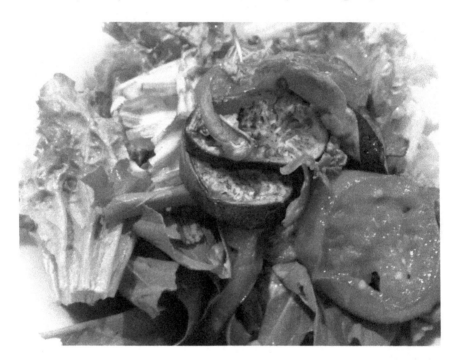

Ingredients

1. 1 eggplant, peeled and diced

1. 1/2 cup water

1. 3 tablespoons vegetable oil

1. 2 cloves garlic, minced

1. 2 cups tomatoes, chopped

1. 1 tablespoon white wine

1. 1 teaspoon cayenne pepper

1. Sea salt and black pepper, to taste

1. 2 tablespoons fresh parsley

Directions

1. Throw the eggplant and water in your pressure cooker. Cover and bring to HIGH pressure; maintain pressure for 4 minutes. Quick release the pressure, remove the lid and set aside.

2. Add the rest of the above ingredients, except for parsley. Bring to HIGHpressure and maintain pressure for about 2 minutes.

3. Sprinkle with fresh parsley and serve chilled.

Country Beef and Potato Stew

(Ready in about 55 minutes | Servings 4)

Ingredients

1. 2 tablespoons olive oil

1. 1 pound beef, cubed

1. 1 small-sized onion, thinly sliced

1. 3 cloves garlic, peeled and minced

1. 4 potatoes, peeled and diced

1. 1 teaspoon dried oregano

1. 1/2 teaspoon dried basil

1. 1 cup tomato sauce

1. 1 cup water

1. 3/4 cup white wine

1. Salt and black pepper, to taste

Directions

1. Warm olive oil in a cooking pot. Sauté the beef, onion, and garlic until themeat has browned and the onion becomes translucent.

2. Add the remaining ingredients; stir to combine ingredients well. Cover andcook for 45 minutes at LOW pressure. Serve over cooked rice and enjoy!

Creamed Beef with Quinoa

(Ready in about 25 minutes | Servings 6)

Ingredients

1. 1 tablespoon olive oil

1. 1 yellow onion, thinly sliced

1. 2 cloves garlic, minced

1. 1 pound top round, cut into strips

1. 1/2 teaspoon cloves, ground

1. 1 teaspoon ground coriander

1. 3/4 teaspoon salt

1. 1/2 teaspoon freshly ground black pepper

1. 1 cup plain yogurt

1. 1 (28-ounce) can whole stewed tomatoes

1. 2 cups prepared quinoa

Directions

1. Heat olive oil in a cooking pot over medium heat. Sauté the onion until tender and translucent. Add the rest of the ingredients, except for quinoa, toyour pressure cooker.

2. Turn the heat up to HIGH; when the cooker reaches pressure, lower theheat. Cook for about 15 minutes at HIGH pressure.

3. Afterwards, open the pressure cooker by releasing pressure. Serve overprepared quinoa.

Saucy Beef in Yogurt

(Ready in about 30 minutes | Servings 6)

Ingredients

1. 1 tablespoon butter, at room temperature
1. 1 red onion, diced
1. 5 green garlics, minced
1. 1 pound bottom round, cubed
1. 1 tablespoon cumin
1. 1 tablespoon coriander
1. 1/2 teaspoon cardamom
1. 1 teaspoon chili powder
1. Salt and black pepper, to taste
1. 2 ripe tomatoes, chopped
1. 1 cup whole milk yogurt

Directions

1. Start by melting the butter over medium heat in your cooker. Sauté theonion and green garlic until they are softened.

2. Add the remaining ingredients, except for the yogurt, to your pressurecooker.

3. Cook for 13 to 15 minutes at HIGH pressure. Lastly, open the cooker byreleasing pressure.

4. Pour in the yogurt; simmer until it has thickened, or 10 to 12 minutes. Servewarm.

Corned Beef and Cabbage

(Ready in about 1 hour | Servings 6)

Ingredients

1. Non-stick cooking spray

1. 2 onions, peeled and sliced

1. 1 corned beef brisket

1. 1 cup apple juice

1. 2 teaspoons orange zest, finely grated

1. 2 teaspoons yellow mustard

1. 1/2 head cabbage, diced

1. Sea salt and ground black pepper, to taste

Directions

1. Treat the inside of the cooker with non-stick cooking spray. Arrange theonions on the bottom of your cooker.

2. Add the beef, apple juice, orange zest, and yellow mustard. Lock the lid into place; bring to LOW pressure; maintain for 45 minutes. Afterwards,remove the lid.

3. Place the cabbage on top of the ingredients. Then, bring to LOW pressure; maintain pressure for 8 minutes. Season with salt and black pepper to taste.

4. Carve the brisket and serve.

DESSERT RECIPES
Winter Steamed Pears
(Ready in about 10 minutes | Servings 4)

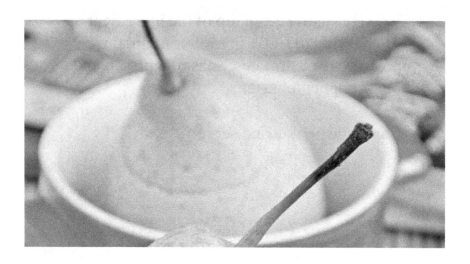

Ingredients

1. 4 pears, cored and halved

1. 1 medium-sized lemon

1. 1/2 teaspoon ground cinnamon

1. 1/2 teaspoon grated nutmeg

1. 1/2 cup water

Directions

1. Drizzle lemon juice over the pears.
   Sprinkle them with cinnamon andnutmeg.

2. Pour the water into the pressure cooker. Place
   a metal rack in the pressurecooker; lay a
   heatproof plate on the rack.

3. Lay the pears on the plate. Cook on HIGH
   pressure for 4 minutes. Turn offthe heat;
   carefully remove the lid.

4. Serve at room temperature or chilled. Garnish
   with some whipped cream if desired.

Ginger Peaches in Syrup

(Ready in about 10 minutes | Servings 6)

Ingredients

1. 2 (15-ounce) cans sliced peaches in syrup

1. 1/4 cup water

1. 1 tablespoon wine vinegar

1. 1/8 teaspoon grated nutmeg

1. 1 teaspoon ground cinnamon

1. 4 whole cloves

1. 1 tablespoon candied ginger, minced

1. A pinch of cayenne pepper

1. Sugar to taste (optional)

Directions

1. Add all the above ingredients to your pressure cooker. Stir to combine. Cover and bring to LOW pressure; maintain pressure for 3 minutes.

2. After that, discard the cloves. Return the pressure cooker to MEDIUM heat;simmer for 5 minutes, stirring frequently.

3. Garnish with a dollop of whipped cream or strawberry ice cream, if desired.Serve immediately or refrigerate before serving.

Coconut Rice Pudding with Pineapple

(Ready in about 10 minutes | Servings 8)

Ingredients

1. 1 cup white rice

1. 1 ½ cups water

1. 1 tablespoon butter, melted

1. 1/4 teaspoon salt

1. 1 (14-ounce) can coconut milk

1. 1/2 cup sugar

1. 2 eggs

1. 1/2 cup milk

1. 1/2 teaspoon allspice

1. 1/2 teaspoon almond extract

1. 1/2 teaspoon vanilla extract

1. 1 can pineapple chunks, well drained

Directions

1. In a pressure cooking pot, combine rice, water, butter, and salt. Lock the lidin place; cook on HIGH and maintain the pressure for 3 minutes.

2. Then, turn off your cooker and use a natural pressure release. Add coconutmilk and sugar; stir to combine well.

3. In a small-sized bowl, whisk the eggs together with milk, allspice, almondextract, and vanilla extract. Pour into your cooker. Then, cook, stirring often, until it starts to boil. Turn off the cooker. Stir in pineapple chunks.

4. Rice pudding will thicken as it cools. Garnish with maraschino cherries andserve chilled.

Winter Apple Dessert

(Ready in about 15 minutes | Servings 6)

Ingredients

1. 6 apples, cored

1. 1 cup red wine

1. 1/4 cup raisins

1. 1/4 cup walnuts, chopped

1. 1/2 cup sugar

1. 1/4 teaspoon grated nutmeg

1. 1/4 teaspoon cardamom

1. 1 teaspoon cinnamon powder

Directions

1. Arrange the apples at the bottom of your pressure cooker. Pour in wine.

2. Then, sprinkle raisins, chopped walnuts, sugar, nutmeg, cardamom, and cinnamon powder. Close and lock the cooker's lid.

3. Cook for 10 minutes at HIGH pressure. Lastly, open the pressure cookerwith the "natural release method".

4. Serve warm or at room temperature. Enjoy!

Hot Chocolate Fondue

(Ready in about 10 minutes | Servings 12)

Ingredients

1. 2 cups water

1. 4 ounces dark chocolate 85%

1. 4 ounces cream

1. 1 teaspoon sugar

1. 1/2 teaspoon cinnamon powder

1. 1/4 teaspoon grated nutmeg

1. 1 teaspoon Amaretto liqueur

Directions

1. Prepare your cooker by adding 2 cups of lukewarm water into the bottom;place trivet and set aside.

2. In a heat-proof container, such as a mug, melt your dark chocolate. Add therest of the above ingredients. Put this container into the pressure cooker. Close and lock the cooker's lid.

3. Cook for 1 to 2 minutes on HIGH pressure. Open the pressure cooker according to manufacturer's directions.

4. Then, pull out the container with tongs. Serve right now with fresh fruits.Enjoy!

INSTANT POT

BREAKFAST RECIPES
Quick and Easy Quinoa
(Ready in about 10 minutes | Servings 6)

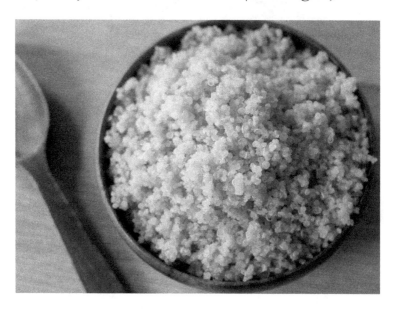

Ingredients

1. 1 cup quinoa, rinsed well

1. 1/2 teaspoon seasoned salt

1. 1/4 teaspoon ground black pepper

1. 1 ½ cups water

1. 1 orange, zested and squeezed

Directions

1. In your cooker, place all the ingredients, except for orange juice.

2. Close and lock the lid. Press "Manual" key and cook for 1 minute. Next, open the cooker using Natural Pressure Release

3. Add orange juice and stir to combine. Taste and adjust for seasonings. Serve.

Mediterranean Wheat Berry Salad

(Ready in about 40 minutes | Servings 6)

Ingredients

1. 1 ½ cups dry wheat berries

1. 2 tablespoons olive oil

1. 4 cups water

1. 1/4 teaspoon sea salt

1. 1 tablespoon olive oil

1. 1 tablespoon apple cider vinegar

1. 1 cup tomatoes, chopped

1. 1/4 cup scallions, chopped

1. 2 ounces feta cheese

1. 1 teaspoon rosemary

Directions

1. Start by toasting the wheat berries.

2. Stir the olive oil into your cooker. Now press the "Sauté" button. Then, addthe toasted wheat berries and cook for 5 minutes, stirring continuously. Press "Cancel".

3. Next, add the water and sea salt; cook under HIGH pressure for 30 minutes.

4. Drain the wheat berries and rinse them with cold water. Place the wheat berries in a salad bowl. Toss with the remaining ingredients. Serve chilled.

Bean and Mint Salad

(Ready in about 10 minutes | Servings 4)

Ingredients

1. 1 cup dry beans, soaked

1. 4 cups water

1. 1 garlic clove, smashed

1. 1 bay leaf

1. 1 sprig fresh mint

1. 2 tablespoons olive oil

1. Sea salt and black pepper, to taste

Directions

1. Add the soaked beans, water, garlic clove, and bay leaf to the cooker.

2. Close and lock the lid. Use "Manual"; choose 8 minutes pressure cookingtime.

3. Use Natural Pressure Release to open the cooker. Strain the beans and transfer to a salad bowl. Toss with the remaining ingredients. Serve chilled.

LUNCH RECIPES
Rainbow Lentil Soup

(Ready in about 20 minutes | Servings 6)

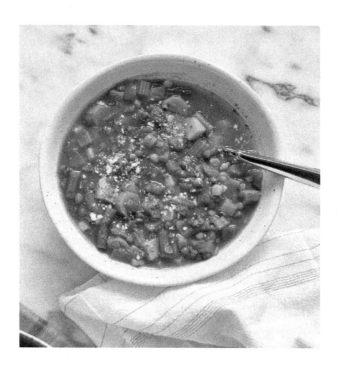

Ingredients

1. 2 cloves garlic, minced

1. 1 red onion, chopped

1. 1 teaspoon smoked paprika

1. Sea salt and ground black pepper, to taste

1. 2 carrots, thinly sliced

1. 1 pound Yukon Gold potatoes, diced

1. 1 cup red lentils, rinsed

1. 1 cup green lentils, rinsed

1. 2 bay leaves

1. 8 cups water

Directions

1. First, choose "Sauté" function. Sauté the garlic, onions, paprika, salt, blackpepper, carrots, and potatoes for about 5 minutes, stirring continuously.

2. Stir in the lentils, bay leaves, and water.

3. Cover the pot and bring to HIGH pressure. Afterwards, use the quick-release method to release the pressure.

4. Taste and adjust the seasonings. Serve warm.

Butternut Squash and Lentil Soup

(Ready in about 20 minutes | Servings 6)

Ingredients

1. 2 tablespoons olive oil

1. 1 onion, diced

1. 3 cloves garlic, minced

1. 1 ½ pounds butternut squash, roughly chopped

1. 1 teaspoon cumin powder

1. 1 teaspoon Garam masala

1. Salt and cayenne pepper to taste

1. 4 cups vegetable stock

1. 1 cup lentils, rinsed

1. 1 can tomatoes, diced

1. Fresh chopped parsley leaves, chopped

Directions

1. Choose the "Sauté" function; warm olive oil. Sauté the onion and garlic for4 to 5 minutes.

2. Add the butternut squash, cumin, Garam masala, salt, and cayenne pepper.Continue to cook for about 3 minutes.

3. Add the stock and lentils. Secure the lid closed. Press the "Manual" button,and adjust the timer to 6 minutes under HIGH pressure. Stir in the tomatoes.

4. Mix the soup with your immersion blender. Serve topped with freshparsley. Enjoy!

Chipotle Pumpkin Soup with Pecans

(Ready in about 25 minutes | Servings 6)

Ingredients

1. 2 cloves garlic, smashed

1. 1 onion, chopped

1. 1 teaspoon ground allspice

1. 1 teaspoon salt

1. 1 teaspoon cayenne pepper

1. 1 teaspoon black pepper

1. 1 chipotle pepper, seeded and finely minced

1. 2 medium-sized potatoes, peeled and diced

1. 2 large apples, peeled, cored and diced

1. 2 (15-ounce) cans pumpkin puree

1. 1/4 cup pecans, pulsed

1. 2 cups water

1. 2 cups vegetable stock

1. Toasted pumpkin seeds, for garnish

Directions

1. Using the "Sauté" function, cook the garlic and onion until they arebrowned, or about 4 minutes.

2. Add allspice, salt, cayenne pepper, black pepper, and chipotle. Add thepotatoes, apples, pumpkin puree, ground pecans, water, and stock.

3. Click the "Manual" button; adjust cooking time to 4 minutes under HIGHpressure. Afterwards, let the pressure release naturally for about 10 minutes.

4. Carefully open the lid; transfer the soup to your food processor; pulse untilcompletely smooth and creamy, working in batches. Serve warm sprinkledwith toasted pumpkin seeds.

DINNER RECIPES
Black Bean and Mango Salad
(Ready in about 15 minutes | Servings 4)

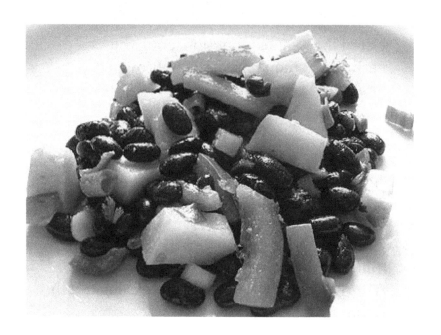

Ingredients

1. 4 cups water

1. 1 cup black beans, soaked overnight

1. 2 bay leaves

1. 1 small-sized mango, diced

1. 1 zucchini, peeled and thinly sliced

1. 1/4 cup cilantro, coarsely chopped

1. 2 tablespoons coconut oil, softened

1. 2 tablespoons lime juice

1. Salt and white pepper, to your liking

Directions

1. Simply put the water, black beans, bay leaves into the inner pot. Choose "Manual" function and 8 minutes pressure cooking time.

2. Drain your beans, discard bay leaves, and allow them to cool completely.Now add the remaining ingredients and stir to combine. Serve right now.

Rice and Tuna Salad

(Ready in about 30 minutes | Servings 4)

Ingredients

1. 2 ½ cups water

1. 2 cups brown rice

1. 2 cups tuna in spring water

1. 1 onion, thinly sliced

1. 1 cup frozen petits pois, defrosted

1. 2 tablespoons extra-virgin olive oil

1. 1 teaspoon red pepper flakes

1. 1/2 teaspoon dried dill weed

1. Salt and ground black pepper, to your liking

1. 1 bunch flat-leaf parsley, roughly chopped

Directions

1. Add lightly salted water and rice to your cooker. Close and lock the lid.Choose "Manual" function and 22 minutes pressure cooking time.

2. Then, open the cooker using natural pressure release. Allow rice to coolcompletely.

3. Add the rest of the ingredients. Stir and serve well chilled.

Peppery Jasmine Rice Salad

(Ready in about 30 minutes | Servings 4)

Ingredients

1. 3 cups Jasmine rice, rinsed

1. 3 cups water

1. 1 green bell pepper, cut into thin strips or chopped

1. 1 red bell pepper, cut into thin strips or chopped

1. 1 orange bell pepper, cut into thin strips or chopped

1. 1 cup scallions, chopped (white and green parts)

1. 1 tablespoon lemon zest, grated

1. 3 tablespoons extra-virgin olive oil

1. 1/3 cup mixed mint and cilantro, roughly chopped

Directions

1. Throw rinsed rice in your Instant Pot. Add water and lock the lid.

2. Press "Manual" key; use the [+ -] button to choose 4 minutes.

3. Next, open the cooker and allow rice to cool completely. Transfer your rice to a salad bowl. Add remaining ingredients. Now stir to combine. Serve andenjoy!

FAST SNACKS
Party Sausage Dip

(Ready in about 15 minutes | Servings 10)

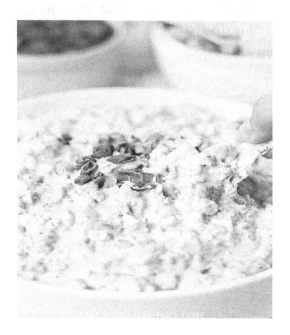

Ingredients

1. 1 tablespoon lard

1. 1 green bell pepper, diced

1. 1 red bell pepper, diced

1. 1 leek, chopped

1. 2 cloves garlic, sliced

1. 1/2 pound ground Italian sausage

1. 1 (28-ounce) can crushed tomatoes

1. 1/4 cup Kalamata olives

1. 1/2 teaspoon red pepper flakes, crushed

1. Salt and ground black pepper to taste

Directions

1. Click "Sauté" and melt the lard. Now sauté bell peppers, leek, and garlic forseveral minutes. Next, stir in sausage and cook until they are just browned.

2. Add the remaining ingredients and cover the pot.

3. Now set cooker's timer for 15 minutes. Release pressure naturally. Servewarm with your favorite dippers.

Meat and Tomato Sauce

(Ready in about 15 minutes | Servings 10)

Ingredients

1. 1 tablespoon olive oil

1. 1 pound lean ground beef

1. 1 pound ground Italian sausage

1. 1 onion, chopped

1. 2 cloves garlic, minced

1. 1/2 cup red wine

1. 2 (28-ounce) cans chopped tomatoes

1. 1 (14-ounce) can chicken broth

1. 1 teaspoon basil

1. 1 teaspoon oregano

1. 1/4 cup heavy cream

Directions

1. Set the cooker on "Sauté" mode; then, warm olive oil and add meat; cooktill it is browned. Reserve 1 tablespoon fat.

2. Stir in the onion and garlic; let them cook for 1 to 2 minutes, stirringconstantly. Deglaze the bottom of your cooker with red wine. Add thecanned tomatoes, chicken broth, basil and oregano.

3. Cover with the lid and set the timer for 8 minutes. Stir in the heavy cream;serve and enjoy.

Buttery Spicy Potatoes

(Ready in about 15 minutes | Servings 8)

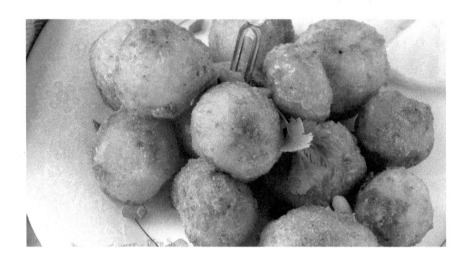

Ingredients

1. 8 red potatoes, diced

1. 3 tablespoons butter

1. 2 tablespoon green garlic, minced

1. Salt and ground black pepper to your liking

1. Fresh chopped cilantro

Directions

1. Put a metal rack into the bottom of your cooker; pour in 1/2 cup of water.

2. Add the potatoes and close the lid; set the timer for 8 minutes. Afterwards,remove the lid carefully. Taste the potatoes for the doneness.

3. Transfer prepared potatoes to a large-sized serving bowl. Toss them withthe remaining ingredients. Enjoy!

DESSERT RECIPES
Baked Apples with Apricots
(Ready in about 15 minutes | Servings 6)

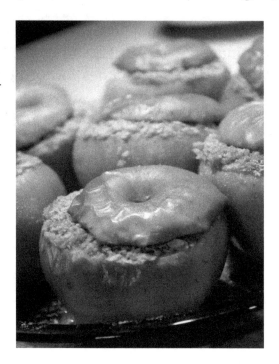

Ingredients

1. 6 apples, cored

1. 1/2 cup dried apricot, chopped

1. 1/2 cup apple brandy

1. 1/2 cup water

1. 2 star anise pods

1. 1/3 cup honey

1. ¼ cup brown sugar

1. 1 teaspoon cinnamon powder

Directions

1. Arrange your apples in the base of the Instant Pot. Add the remaining ingredients.

2. Select "Manual" and set the time to 10 minutes. Perform Natural releasemethod.

3. Serve dolloped with whipped cream. Enjoy!

Poached Figs with Yogurt Cream

(Ready in about 15 minutes | Servings 4)

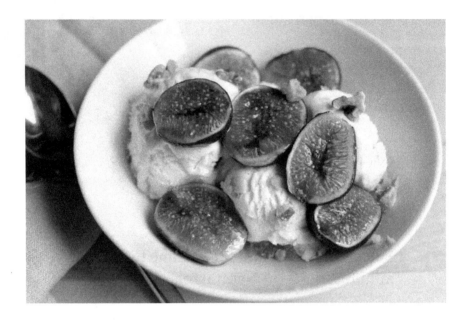

Ingredients

1. 1 pound figs

1. 1 cup red wine

1. 1/2 cup honey

1. 1/2 teaspoon grated nutmeg

1. 1/2 cup almonds, toasted and roughly chopped

Directions

1. Arrange the figs in the bottom of your cooker. Add the rest of the ingredients.

2. Cover and select "Manual" mode. Now set the timer to 9 minutes pressurecooking time. Use Normal Release method.

3. Serve with yogurt cream and enjoy!

Cinnamon Bread Pudding with Figs

(Ready in about 15 minutes | Servings 6)

Ingredients

1. 2 cups water

1. 1 teaspoon coconut oil, at room temperature

1. 4 cups stale sweet cinnamon bread, cubed

1. 2 cups almond milk

1. 3 whole eggs, beaten

1. 1/2 cup dried figs, chopped

1. 1/2 teaspoon grated nutmeg

1. 1/2 ground cloves

1. 1 teaspoon cinnamon powder

1. 1/4 teaspoon salt

1. 1/4 teaspoon almond extract

1. 1/2 teaspoon vanilla paste

Directions

1. Pour the water into the Instant Pot. Place the steam rack on the bottom.

2. Grease a casserole dish with coconut oil. Add bread cubes to the casseroledish.

3. In a mixing bowl, combine the rest of the ingredients. Pour the mixture overbread cubes. Cover with wax paper or an aluminum foil.

4. Select "Steam" mode and adjust the timer to 15 minutes. Serve warm or atroom temperature.

CPSIA information can be obtained
at www.ICGtesting.com
Printed in the USA
BVHW040347190521
607637BV00005BA/887

9 781802 892420